Vegan Diet

5 Ingredients or Less - Quick, Easy, & Healthy Vegetarian Plant Based Recipes

(Weight Loss And All Day Energy)

Ian Lara

Published by Robert Satterfield Publishing House

© **Ian Lara**

All Rights Reserved

Vegan Diet Cookbook: 5 Ingredients or Less - Quick, Easy, & Healthy Vegetarian Plant Based Recipes (Weight Loss And All Day Energy)

ISBN 978-1-989682-92-0

All rights reserved. No part of this guide may be reproduced in any form without permission in writing from the publisher except in the case of brief quotations embodied in critical articles or reviews.

Legal & Disclaimer

The information contained in this book is not designed to replace or take the place of any form of medicine or professional medical advice. The information in this book has been provided for educational and entertainment purposes only.

The information contained in this book has been compiled from sources deemed reliable, and it is accurate to the best of the Author's knowledge; however, the Author cannot guarantee its accuracy and validity and cannot be held liable for any errors or omissions. Changes are periodically made to this book. You must consult your doctor or get professional medical advice before using any of the suggested remedies, techniques, or information in this book.

TABLE OF CONTENT

Part 1 1

Introduction.. 2

Delicious Vegan Recipes 5

Recipes Included In This Book 5

Vegan Recipes 7

Berry Beet Smoothie 7

Cool And Refreshing Watermelon Smoothie 8

Banana Chai Smoothie 9

Green Power Smoothie 10

Mixed Fruits Beet Juice 10

Cranberry Salad With White Wine Vinegar 11

Broccoli Almond Salad... 12

Paprika Spinach Salad With Strawberries 13

Tomato Salad With Balsamic Vinegar And Feta Cheese..... 15

Apple Salad With Mustard And Maple Syrup..................... 16

Peanut Butter Rice With Tofu 17

Vegetarian Potato Hummus............................... 19

Miso Soup With Avocado And Shiitake Mushrooms.......... 20

Green Pea Soup In Almond Milk......................... 22

Coconut Banana Pudding 22

Tofu And Soymilk Vanilla Cheesecake................................ 23

- Pineapple And Orange Lemon Sorbet 24
- Banana Vanilla And Chocolate Dessert Pudding 26
- Watermelon Lime And Vanilla Ice Pops 27
- Part 2 28
- Introduction.. 29
- Herbal Green Pea 30
- Spicy Cucumber Cabbage 30
- Mexican Fiesta.. 31
- Sea Soup Specialty... 31
- Tomato Basil... 32
- Cream Of Cucumber 32
- Cream Of Tomato 32
- Cream Of Nectarine... 33
- Cream Of Mango 33
- Cream Of Carrot 34
- Green Goodness 34
- Fennel Basil Tomato Soup 34
- Cream Of Lime... 35
- Cream Of Celery 35
- Cream Of Zucchini 36
- Cream Of Pumpkin 36
- Green Onion Tomato Soup... 37

Cream Of Spinach 37

Carrot Ginger Soup 37

Cream Of Broccoli 38

Garden Blend 38

Cream Of Cauliflower 39

Strawberry Beet Soup 39

Spicy Lime Soup 40

Carrot Soup 40

Cream Of Lemon 41

Cream Of Mushroom 41

Cream Of Cabbage 41

Cream Of Pumpkin 42

Winter Specialty Soup 42

Thai Ginger Soup 43

Cooling Watermelon Soup 44

Vegan Heaven Soup 44

Light Lettuce Soup 44

Belly Buster Soup 45

Cream Of Pepper 45

Wonderland Soup 46

Cream Of Chestnut 46

Exquisite Tomato Soup 46

Cream Of Corn 47

About The Author 48

Part 1

Introduction

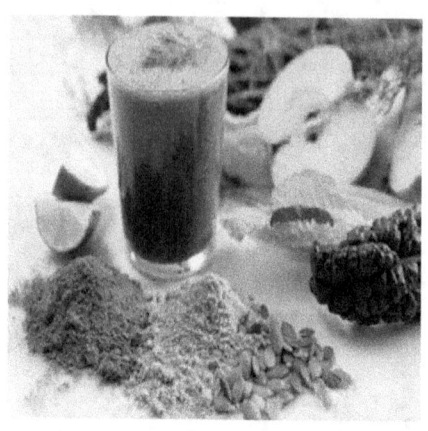

A vegan or vegetarian diet consists of only plant-based foods. Vegan meals and recipes do not incorporate meat, dairy products, eggs or any other types of food that are of animal origin. Going vegan does not mean that you need to eat whole fruits and vegetables. In fact, chips, French fries, doughnuts, ice cream and other types of food can be considered vegan if instead of butter, they are made with vegetable oil. Vegan meals and recipes are one of the healthiest ways to eat. If you decide to try this diet, make sure that you choose only plant-based foods. These are fruits and vegetables, whole grains, nuts, beans, lentils and seeds. They have high amounts of antioxidants and are loaded with vitamins, nutrients, minerals, fiber and healthy oils that the body needs. To get enough protein, you can get it from grains and soy together with beans.

Following this diet will allow you to get all the vitamins and nutrients that you need while limiting your intake of sugar, calories, salt, trans fats and other preservatives that can harm the body. There are many benefits that being a vegan offers. First, it is much healthier compared to the common, average diets of many individuals. Vegetarian recipes use ingredients with no animal fat and cholesterol and focus more on incorporating fruits and vegetables, which are loaded with many antioxidants that can prevent and reverse diseases, as well as reduce your risk of getting certain types of cancer. The second benefit is going vegan will help control weight. Many types of food contain trans fats and preservatives that make people fat and unhealthy. However, vegan recipes are low-fat and contain good doses of sugar and carbohydrates, which will still provide you with energy to last throughout the day without feeling hungry.

People who eat lots of fruits and vegetables are proven to live longer than those who love eating different types of food which contain animal fat. Animal-based food products can really clog the body's arteries, make you gain weight and even providing you with less energy. The benefits of going vegan go beyond your own health. For some people, going vegan is simply not for health reasons but for environmental reasons as well. Eating fruits and vegetables can lessen industrial farms, which can in turn lessen the number of polluted rivers and lands. Aside from that, you will save much more money if you buy plant-based ingredients instead of using meat and dairy products, as they are a lot cheaper.

Many people are afraid to go on the vegan diet because of the notion that vegan recipes are not delicious because of their lack of flavor. On the contrary, though, it is so much easier to go vegan these days, as there are a lot of absolutely delicious vegan recipes available—from smoothies to salads to entrees to desserts—that you won't even realize they are vegan. So, instead of thinking of reasons as to why you should go on a vegan diet, what you should think about is why you haven't gone vegan.

Delicious Vegan Recipes

Recipes Included in This Book

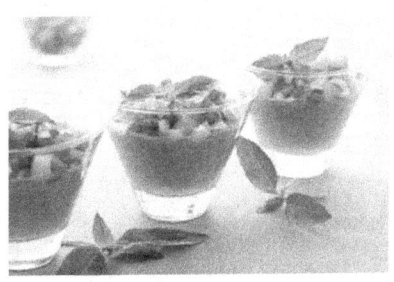

Berry Beet Smoothie
Cool and Refreshing Watermelon Smoothie
Banana Chai Smoothie
Green Power Smoothie
Mixed Fruits Beet Juice
Cranberry Salad with White Wine Vinegar
Broccoli Almond Salad
Paprika Spinach Salad with Strawberries
Tomato Salad with Balsamic Vinegar and Feta Cheese
Apple Salad with Mustard and Maple Syrup
Peanut Butter Rice with Tofu
Sunflower and Basil Pesto Pasta
Vegetarian Potato Hummus
Miso Soup with Avocado and Shitake Mushrooms
Green Pea Soup in Almond Milk
Coconut Banana Pudding
Tofu and Soy Milk Vanilla Cheesecake
Pineapple and Orange Lemon Sorbet
Banana Vanilla and Chocolate Dessert Pudding

Watermelon Lime and Vanilla Ice Pops

Vegan Recipes

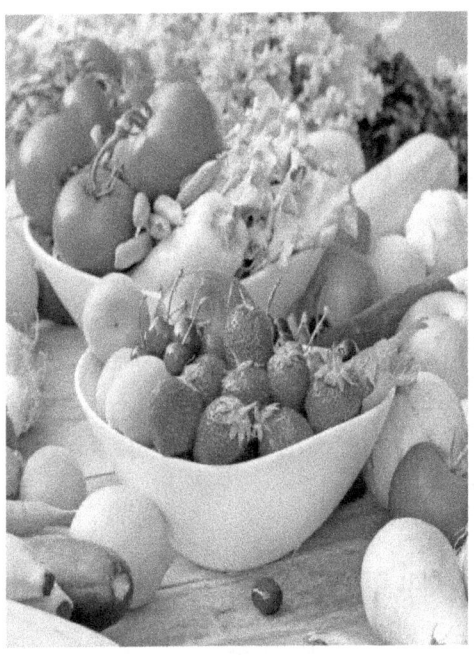

Berry Beet Smoothie

Prep Time: 5 minutes
Servings: 1

Ingredients:

1 cup of water
6 strawberries
2 slices of raw red beet, chopped
15 green grapes
½ cucumber, peeled
½ orange, skin removed
2 large handfuls of spinach
4-6 ice cubes

Directions:

1. Place all ingredients in the blender and process until smooth.
2. Pour in 2 glasses and serve immediately.

Cool and Refreshing Watermelon Smoothie

Prep Time: 5 minutes
Servings: 1

Ingredients:

2 cups of cubed watermelon, seeded
5 strawberries
½ cup of coconut water

Directions:

1. Place all ingredients in the blender and process until smooth.
2. Pour in a glass and serve immediately.

Banana Chai Smoothie

Prep Time: 5 minutes
Servings: 1

Ingredients:

1 cup of unsweetened almond milk
1 medium ripe banana, sliced
1 teaspoon of coconut butter
½ teaspoon of chai spice
1 knob of fresh ginger, peeled

Directions:

1. Place all ingredients in the blender and process until smooth.
1. Pour in a glass and serve immediately.

Green Power Smoothie

Prep Time: 5 minutes
Servings: 1

Ingredients:

10 ounces of brewed green tea
1 cup of cubed honeydew melon
1 plum, pitted
20 green grapes
½ cucumber, peeled and sliced
1 large handful of spinach
3-4 ice cubes

Directions:

1. Place all ingredients in the blender and process until smooth.
2. Pour in a glass and serve immediately.

Mixed Fruits Beet Juice

Prep Time: 5 minutes
Servings: 1

Ingredients:

2/3 cup of apple juice
3 tablespoons of beet juice
1 cup of mixed berries
½ banana

Directions:

1. Place all ingredients in the blender and process until smooth.
2. Pour in a glass and serve immediately.

Cranberry Salad with White Wine Vinegar

Prep Time: 15 minutes
Servings: 18

Ingredients:

3 cups of chopped broccoli
3 cups of chopped cauliflower

3 cups of chopped celery
1 10-ounce package of frozen peas, thawed
1 cup of sweetened dried cranberries
1 ½ cups of mayonnaise
¼ cup of Parmesan cheese
¼ cup of white sugar
2 tablespoons of grated onion
1 tablespoon of white wine vinegar
1 teaspoon of salt
1 cup of Spanish peanuts

Directions:

1. In a large bowl, mix together broccoli, cauliflower, celery peas and cranberries.
2. In a separate bowl, whisk together mayonnaise, cheese, sugar, onion, white wine vinegar and salt.
3. Pour salad dressing over the vegetables and sprinkle peanuts on top.

Broccoli Almond Salad

Prep Time: 15 minutes

Servings: 8-10

Ingredients:

2 heads of fresh broccoli
1 red onion
¾ cup of raisins
¾ cup of sliced almonds
1 cup of mayonnaise
½ cup of white sugar
2 tablespoons of white wine vinegar

Directions:

1. Chop broccoli into bite-size pieces and the onions into thin slices.
2. Combine broccoli, onions, raisins and almonds in a bowl.
3. In a separate bowl, whisk the mayonnaise, white sugar and white wine vinegar together.
4. Pour salad dressing over the broccoli and serve.

Paprika Spinach Salad with Strawberries

Prep Time: 10 minutes
Servings: 8

Ingredients:

2 bunches of spinach, cut into bite-sized pieces
4 cups of strawberries, sliced
½ cup of vegetable oil
¼ cup of white wine vinegar
½ cup of white sugar
¼ teaspoon of paprika
2 tablespoons of sesame seeds
1 tablespoon of poppy seeds

Directions:

1. Mix spinach and strawberries in a large bowl.
2. In a separate bowl, combine vegetable oil, white wine vinegar, sugar, paprika, sesame seeds and poppy seeds together.
3. Pour salad dressing over spinach and strawberries and serve.

Tomato Salad with Balsamic Vinegar and Feta Cheese

Prep Time: 15 minutes
Servings: 4

Ingredients:

6 Roma tomatoes, diced
1 small cucumber, peeled and chopped
3 green onions, chopped
¼ cup of fresh basil leaves, cut into strips
3 tablespoons of olive oil
2 tablespoons of balsamic vinegar
3 tablespoons of crumbled feta cheese
Salt to taste
Pepper to taste

Directions:

1. Toss all ingredients together in a large bowl.
2. Season with salt and pepper.

Apple Salad with Mustard and Maple Syrup

Prep Time: 20 minutes
Servings: 2

Ingredients:

2 Granny Smith apples, peeled, cored and sliced
½ lemon, juiced
6 cups of thinly sliced kale
½ avocado, thinly sliced
¼ cup of chopped almonds
½ cup of olive oil
¼ cup of apple cider vinegar
2 tablespoons of maple syrup
2 teaspoons of grainy mustard
1 teaspoon of ground black pepper
½ teaspoon of kosher salt

Directions:

1. Coat apples with lemon juice in a bowl and add the kale, avocado and almonds.
2. In a separate bowl, mix together olive oil, apple cider vinegar, maple syrup, grainy mustard, ground black pepper and kosher salt.
3. Pour over salad and serve.

Peanut Butter Rice with Tofu

Prep Time: 15 minutes
Servings: 2

Ingredients:

2 ½ cups of cooked brown rice
1 ¼ cups of cubed tofu
1 teaspoon of cilantro
1 teaspoon of chopped peanuts
3 tablespoons of peanut butter
1 tablespoon of lime juice
2 ½ teaspoons of agave syrup
¾ cup of water
3 teaspoons of soy sauce
2 teaspoons of olive oil

Directions:

1. Place peanut butter, lime juice, agave syrup, water and soy sauce in a blender or a food processor. Process until smooth. Transfer to a bowl.
2. Heat olive oil in a pan over low-medium heat and sauté tofu for about 3 minutes.
3. Add tofu in the peanut butter sauce and mix well to coat. Transfer tofu to a plate.
4. Add the cooked rice in the remaining peanut butter sauce and mix.
5. Transfer rice to a serving dish and place tofu on top.
6. Sprinkle with cilantro and chopped peanuts.
7. Sunflower and Basil Pesto Pasta

Prep Time: 20 minutes
Servings: 6-8

Ingredients:

2 pounds of pasta (your choice of pasta)
½ cup of lemon juice
4 cloves of garlic, minced
1/3 cup of extra virgin olive oil
1 bunch of fresh basil leaves
1 cup of raw spinach
1 small jalapeno, with seeds
1 tablespoon of maple syrup
¾ cup of raw sunflowers
½ cup of almonds, crushed
Salt to taste
Pepper to taste

Directions:

1. Cook pasta according to the package instructions. Drain and transfer to a serving dish.
2. While pasta is cooking, add the rest of the ingredients in a blender or a food processor and process until smooth.
3. Pour pasta sauce all over pasta and serve immediately.

Vegetarian Potato Hummus

Prep Time: 10 minutes
Servings: 1

Ingredients:

2 slices of whole-wheat sourdough, toasted
1 cup of oven-baked sweet potato
1 ½ cups of garbanzo beans
2 tablespoons of apple cider vinegar
2 tablespoons of tahini
4 tablespoons of grape seed oil
2 teaspoons of agave syrup
¼ cup of lemon juice

Directions:

1. Place all ingredients except for the bread in the blender and process until smooth.
2. Slather hummus on bread and serve.

Miso Soup with Avocado and Shiitake

Mushrooms

Prep Time: 10 minutes
Servings: 2

Ingredients:

1 Portobello mushroom
½ avocado
2 tablespoons of miso
2 cups of hot water
1 teaspoon of walnut oil
3 sliced shitake mushrooms plus 3 more unsliced
Salt to taste
Pepper to taste
¼ cup of fresh cilantro leaves

Directions:

1. Place all ingredients except for the 3 sliced shiitake mushrooms and cilantro leaves in the blender and process until smooth.
2. Season with salt and pepper.
3. Pour soup into bowls and sprinkle each bowl with shiitake mushrooms and cilantro leaves.

Green Pea Soup in Almond Milk

Prep Time: 10 minutes
Servings: 2

Ingredients:

2 cups of green peas
1 avocado, peeled, pitted and chopped
1 ½ cups of almond milk
1 small onion
1 teaspoon of salt
½ teaspoon of pepper

Directions:

1. Place 1 cup of peas in a blender and add in the avocado, almond milk, onion, salt and pepper. Process until smooth.
2. Pour into bowls and top soup with the remaining green peas.

Coconut Banana Pudding

Prep Time: 10 minutes
Servings: 4

Ingredients:

1 avocado, peeled, pitted and cut into chunks
1 banana, peeled and cut into chunks
1 cup of unsweetened soymilk
¼ cup of raw cocoa powder
2 tablespoons of agave nectar
1 teaspoon of lemon juice
¼ cup of shredded, unsweetened coconut

Directions:

1. Place all the ingredients in a blender and process until smooth.
2. Pour into an airtight container and let set in the refrigerator for an hour before serving.

Tofu and Soymilk Vanilla Cheesecake

Prep Time: 15 minutes
Servings: 6

Ingredients:

1 12 oz. package of soft tofu
½ cup of soymilk
½ cup of white sugar
1 tablespoon of vanilla extract
¼ cup of maple syrup
1 9-inch graham cracker crust

Directions:

1. Preheat oven to 350 degrees F.
2. Place tofu, soymilk, white sugar, vanilla extract and maple syrup in a blender and process until smooth. Pour mixture into the graham cracker crust.
3. Bake cheesecake in the preheated oven for 30 minutes.
4. Remove from the oven and allow to cool completely.
5. When cool, let cake set in the refrigerator for at least 2 hours before serving.

Pineapple and Orange Lemon Sorbet

Prep Time: 20 minutes
Servings: 10

Ingredients:

½ cup of water
½ cup of granulated sugar
2 cups of orange juice
1 tablespoon of lemon juice
1 20-ounce can of crushed pineapple

Directions:

1. Heat a saucepan over medium heat and add water and sugar. Bring to a simmer until sugar is completely dissolved.
2. Puree pineapple with its juice in a blender until smooth. Transfer to a large bowl and add in the sugar syrup, orange juice and lemon juice. Place bowl in the freezer until slightly solid but not totally frozen.
3. Pour mixture again in the blender and process until smooth.

4. Transfer mixture to an airtight container and place in the freezer for 2 hours before serving.

Banana Vanilla and Chocolate Dessert

Pudding

Prep Time: 5 minutes
Servings: 2

Ingredients:

1 banana, peeled and sliced
2 cups of silken tofu
1/3 cup of cocoa powder
1/3 cup of sugar
2 teaspoons of vanilla extract

Directions:

1. Place all ingredients in the blender and process until smooth.
2. Pour into an airtight container and place in the refrigerator. Let set for an hour before serving.

Watermelon Lime and Vanilla Ice Pops

Prep Time: 15 minutes
Servings: 8

Ingredients:

2 ½ cups of chopped watermelon, seeded
1 teaspoon of vanilla extract
2 tablespoons of lime juice
1 tablespoon of food-grade rosewater

Directions:

1. Place all ingredients the blender and process until smooth.
2. Pour into popsicle trays and place in the freezer for 3-4 hours or until frozen.

Part 2

Introduction

First off, all of these recipes would be impossible to make without a blender. All soups serve 1 to 3 people. Feel free to garnish with your favorite dried or fresh herbs, soaked nuts, diced vegetables, or fruit. Out of the listed ingredients for each soup you can choose not to blend the ones you want to save for your garnish. If your heart desires a warm soup then you can lightly heat over the stove, use hot water in the recipe, or blend using the soup mode on your high speed blender. Aside from tasting better, being better for your body, and being cruelty-free; uncooked vegan soups take less prep time. I personally love these recipes and use one or more every day. Raw soups are so beneficial for the human body because they practically digest themselves. Raw food is anything that isn't heated over 118 degrees so that the precious enzymes aren't destroyed. In order for food to digest it must be broken down by enzymes. Science has recently discovered that our bodies can only produce so many enzymes in this lifetime which is the number one reason to eat as much raw food as you enjoy. A great way to start is by trying the soups!

Herbal Green Pea
- 2 cups peas
- 1 avocado
- 1 ½ cups almond milk
- ½ cup fresh basil
- ½ small red onion
- ½ cup fresh chives
- 1 clove garlic
- sea salt to taste

Spicy Cucumber Cabbage
- 2 large cucumbers
- 3 cabbage leaves
- 1 (hot) pepper of choice
- 1 small heirloom tomato
- 2 tablespoons olive oil
- pink Himalayan salt to taste

Mexican Fiesta

- 2 medium heirloom tomatoes
- 2 red bell peppers
- 8 sun dried tomatoes
- 8 sprigs of fresh cilantro
- 2 stalks celery
- 1 cup water
- fresh squeeze lime juice
- ½ avocado
- 2 tbsp. cold-pressed olive oil
- 1 clove garlic
- ¼ tsp. cumin
- ½ tsp. chili or cayenne powder
- ½ teaspoon paprika
- sea salt to taste

Sea Soup Specialty

- 3 cups zucchini noodles made with spiralizer (add in whole after soup is blended)
- 3 nori sheets
- 1 tsp. dulse
- ½ tsp. kelp granules

- 2 tbsp. coconut oil
- 2 cups hot water or your favorite tea

Tomato Basil

- 3 medium heirloom tomatoes
- 4 sun dried tomatoes
- 2 stalks celery
- small chunk of red onion
- ½ clove fresh garlic
- 5 leaves fresh basil
- ½ avocado
- sea salt to taste

Cream of Cucumber

- 2 large cucumbers (peel and all if organic)
- ½ cup macadamia nuts
- squeeze of fresh lemon juice
- 1 clove garlic
- 1 avocado
- 1 cup of water
- sea salt to taste

Cream of Tomato

- 2 large heirloom tomatoes
- 3 stalks celery
- 1 medium carrot
- 1 clove garlic
- juice of 1 lemon
- ½ cup raw cashews
- 1 avocado
- 1 orange bell pepper
- 2 pitted dried medjool dates (optional)
- ½ tsp. cumin
- 5 sprigs cilantro
- 1 tbsp. soaked pumpkin seeds
- pink Himalayan salt to taste

Cream of Nectarine
- 7 to 8 peeled and pitted nectarines (depending on size)
- 2 cups spinach
- ½ cup water
- ½ tsp. cinnamon

Cream of Mango
- 3 cups fresh mango
- 1 cup coconut milk

- 1 tbsp. coconut cream
- 2 tbsp. coconut sugar
- 3 leaves fresh mint
- 3 leaves fresh spearmint

Cream of Carrot

- 2 large carrots
- 1 cup macadamia nuts
- 1 clove garlic
- 1 tbsp. raw apple cider vinegar
- 3 green onions
- 1 red bell pepper
- sea salt to taste

Green Goodness

- 1 cucumber (peel and all if organic)
- 1 cup spinach
- 1 orange bell pepper
- 1 avocado
- 1 tbsp. raw tahini
- juice of 1 lemon
- sea salt to taste

Fennel Basil Tomato Soup

- 1 fennel bulb
- 1 cup water
- 2 medium heirloom tomatoes
- ½ cup fresh basil
- ½ yellow bell pepper
- fresh squeeze lime juice
- sea salt to taste

Cream of Lime

- 2 avocados
- juice of 2 small limes (or 1 large)
- 3 sprigs fresh cilantro
- ½ cup fresh chives
- 1 tsp. cumin
- 1 stalk celery
- 1 cup water
- sea salt to taste

Cream of Celery

- 7 stalks celery
- ½ cup raw cashews
- 1 avocado
- 1 clove garlic

- 1 cup water
- kala namak salt to taste

Cream of Zucchini

- 3 cups zucchini (peel and all if organic)
- 1 cup peas
- 2 stalks celery
- 1 avocado
- 1 cup water
- juice of 1 lemon
- 2 cloves fresh garlic
- 1 tsp. fresh thyme
- 1 tsp. turmeric
- pinch of cayenne pepper
- sea salt to taste

Cream of Pumpkin

- 1 cup pumpkin (seeds and skin removed)
- 2 pitted dried medjool dates
- 1 cup raw cashews
- ¼ tsp. cinnamon
- sea salt to taste

Green Onion Tomato Soup

- 2 large heirloom tomatoes
- 1 yellow bell pepper
- 3 green onions
- 1 cucumber
- 1 clove garlic
- ½ small red onion
- sea salt to taste

Cream of Spinach

- 2 cups spinach
- 1 cup water
- 1 cup macadamia nuts
- 4 green onions
- 1 clove garlic
- ½ tsp nutmeg
- sea salt to taste

Carrot Ginger Soup

- 2 large carrots
- 1 thumb-sized piece of ginger
- 2 tbsp. black sesame seeds

- 2 pitted dried medjool dates
- pinch of black or cayenne pepper
- ½ tsp. turmeric
- 2 cups water
- sea salt to taste

Cream of Broccoli

- 1 head of broccoli (excluding stalk)
- 2 stalks celery
- 1 clove garlic
- ½ small red onion
- fresh squeeze lemon juice
- tsp. dried oregano
- 1 cup water
- pinch of black pepper
- ½ tsp turmeric
- kala namak salt to taste

Garden Blend

- 1 zucchini (peel and all if organic)
- 2 medium heirloom tomatoes
- 2 stalks celery
- 2 medium carrots
- 1 clove garlic

- 2 pitted dried medjool dates
- 1 cup water
- 2 tbsp. olive oil
- pinch of black pepper
- 1 tsp. turmeric
- sea salt to taste

Cream of Cauliflower
- 4 cups cauliflower
- 1 cup soaked raw almonds
- 1 tsp. olive oil
- 1 tsp. coconut oil
- 1 cup arugula
- ½ tsp. rosemary
- sea salt to taste

Strawberry Beet Soup
- 10 whole strawberries (including green tops)
- 2 small beets
- 2 cups water
- 3 green onions
- sea salt to taste

Spicy Lime Soup

- 1 stalk celery
- 1 cup yellow squash
- juice of 1 lime
- 1 chili pepper
- 2 medium carrots
- 2 small heirloom tomatoes
- 1 cup zucchini
- 1 cup cabbage
- 1 clove garlic
- 1 cup water
- sea salt to taste

Carrot Soup

- 1 whole head of broccoli
- 2 medium carrots
- 1 medium heirloom tomato
- ½ zucchini
- 5 raw brazil nuts
- 1 cup water
- sea salt to taste

Cream of Lemon

- 1 lemon (peel and all if organic)
- 1 small heirloom tomato
- 1 avocado
- ¼ cup olive oil
- ½ cup fresh parsley
- 4 stalks celery
- 1 tsp. maple syrup
- 3 cups water
- sea salt to taste

Cream of Mushroom

- 8 oz. of your favorite mushrooms
- 2 cups water
- 4 green onions
- ½ cup cashews
- ¼ cup pine nuts
- ¼ cup hazelnuts
- 4 sprigs fresh parsley
- sea salt to taste

Cream of Cabbage

- 2 cups cabbage

- 2 cups peas
- 1 avocado
- ½ zucchini (peel and all if organic)
- 1 stalk celery
- 1 tbsp. chia seeds
- ½ small red onion
- sea salt to taste

Cream of Pumpkin

- 2 cups pumpkin
- 2 cups water
- 2 cups cauliflower
- ½ cup pecans
- ½ tsp. mustard powder
- 1 tsp. cumin
- 3 sprigs cilantro
- sea salt to taste

Winter Specialty Soup

- 2 cups water
- 3 cups pumpkin
- 1 small carrot
- 2 green onions

- 1 stalk celery
- 1 cup kale
- 1 thumb-sized chunk of ginger
- 1 clove garlic
- 1 avocado
- 1 chili pepper
- sea salt to taste

Thai Ginger Soup
- 2 cups water
- ½ red bell pepper
- 1 small carrot
- 1 stalk celery
- 1 acorn squash
- 3 green onions
- fresh squeeze lemon juice
- 1 small apple
- ½ cup cashews
- 1 thumb-sized chunk of ginger
- 1 clove garlic
- 3 sprigs cilantro
- sea salt to taste

Cooling Watermelon Soup

- 3 cups watermelon
- juice of 1 lime
- 1 small cucumber (peel and all if organic)
- ½ cup fresh mint

Vegan Heaven Soup

- 2 cups water
- 2 cups broccoli
- 2 stalks celery
- 2 green onions
- ½ cup cashews
- 1 clove garlic
- 1 sprig fresh rosemary
- 1 sprig fresh lime
- sea salt to taste

Light Lettuce Soup

- ½ lb. romaine lettuce
- 2 cups peas
- 2 green onions
- 1 cup water
- sea salt to taste

Belly Buster Soup

- 1 small raw sweet potato
- 2 cups water
- 1 cup pumpkin
- 1 red bell pepper
- 1 stalk celery
- 1 medium carrot
- 1 green onion
- 1 small heirloom tomato
- 1 cup cabbage
- sea salt to taste

Cream of Pepper

- 1 red bell pepper
- 1 clove garlic
- 1 avocado
- 1 large heirloom tomato
- ½ small red onion
- 1 tsp. cumin
- sea salt to taste

Wonderland Soup

- 2 cups swiss chard
- 3 cups water
- 1 small carrot
- 1 stalk celery
- 2 green onions
- ½ cup brazil nuts
- 1 clove garlic
- squeeze of fresh lime juice
- ½ tsp. turmeric
- pinch of black pepper
- sea salt to taste

Cream of Chestnut

- 2 cups water
- ½ cup chestnuts
- 2 large carrots
- 1 stalk celery
- 1 sprig of parsley, rosemary and thyme
- 2 basil leaves
- sea salt to taste

Exquisite Tomato Soup

- 1 cup brazil nut milk

- 1 cup water
- 1 large heirloom tomato
- ½ cup sun dried tomatoes
- 1 red bell pepper
- 1 stalk celery
- ½ small red onion
- ¼ cup cashews
- 1 small carrot
- ¼ cup fresh basil
- 1 clove garlic
- pinch of cayenne pepper
- 1 tsp. oregano
- 2 tbsps. lemon juice
- sea salt to taste

Cream of Corn

- 2 cups raw corn
- ¼ cup cashews
- 1 cup water
- 1 clove garlic
- sea salt to taste

About the Author

Ian Lara is author of several cookbooks on Vegan diet. He has written research papers on the topic and currently lives in California.

www.ingramcontent.com/pod-product-compliance
Lightning Source LLC
LaVergne TN
LVHW020439080526
838202LV00055B/5265